Sam C

over

come

DON'T

over-

think

How to Ease Anxiety and Stop
Worry Taking Over Your Life

OVERCOME DON'T OVERTHINK

An Hachette UK Company
www.hachette.co.uk

Vie Books, an imprint of Summersdale Publishers
Part of Octopus Publishing Group Limited
Carmelite House
50 Victoria Embankment
LONDON
EC4Y 0DZ
UK

www.summersdale.com

Printed and bound in China

ISBN: 978-1-83799-351-2

Substantial discounts on bulk quantities of Summersdale books are available to corporations, professional associations and other organizations. For details contact general enquiries: telephone: +44 (0) 1243 771107 or email: enquiries@summersdale.com.

Disclaimer
Neither the author nor the publisher can be held responsible for any injury, loss or claim – be it health, financial or otherwise – arising out of the use, or misuse, of the suggestions made herein. This book is not intended as a substitute for the medical advice of a doctor or physician. If you are experiencing problems with your physical or mental health, it is always best to follow the advice of a medical professional.

Contents

Introduction

We all have times when we worry. Whether you've got some tricky exams looming, or you're concerned about someone you care about, life is full of the kinds of ups and downs that we somehow manage to tackle with aplomb and come out smiling from. But sometimes life presents a problem that makes us worry *too much*. We start imagining worst-case scenarios and dwelling on the things we *should* have done but didn't. Instead of overcoming the challenge, we start overthinking it instead.

But the good news is that you *can* tackle life's challenges without worry – hurrah! In this book, you'll find a mix of ideas, tips and techniques to help you develop a toolkit for when overthinking becomes overwhelming.

Facing your anxieties head-on is never easy, but picking up this book means that you're one step closer to freeing up headspace for positivity instead.

Sound good? Great, let's get started!

No amount of regretting can change the past, and no amount of worrying can change the future.

Roy T. Bennett

1
What is Overthinking?

Whether it's worrying about what *could* happen, or ruminating on what *did* happen, our ability to think critically – about situations or about ourselves – can be a double-edged sword. Spending time in our own heads can sometimes be insightful, but if it's interfering with our ability to take action when we hit an obstacle then it's probably doing more harm than good.

Before we start tackling our overthinking habits, it can be useful to understand why we overthink in the first place. Read on to find out why your worries might have gone rogue, and what that looks like for you.

Are you an overthinker?

Humans are hardwired to think – fact. Our ability to ruminate and reflect is what distinguishes us from all other species on planet Earth. It's a skill that has allowed us to send astronauts to the moon and to cure diseases (as well as do important things such as remembering to take a coat when it looks like rain, or be able to fix a broken shelf before the whole lot falls down).

The problem is that sometimes we convince ourselves that thinking about something for a long time – especially something we perceive to be a problem – is the key to working out the solution. In reality, all we're doing is draining mental energy away from the part of the brain that wants us to be productive and solve the problem. And when we get into a spiral of overthinking, it makes it hard for us to focus on anything else. Annoyingly, it then becomes our default setting whenever we're finding something difficult, and, before we know it, we've inadvertently created a negative mental habit – thanks, brain!

On the next page you'll find some signs of overthinking that may sound a little familiar...

What does overthinking look like?

Overthinking can present itself in lots of ways, and your experience might be entirely different to the next person's. It can also make us react to situations differently and affect our behaviour too. Here are some of the most common signs that you're overthinking things:

~ Thinking about a problem so much that you start to neglect other areas of your life

~ Thinking of all the worst-case scenarios

~ Finding it difficult to relax

~ A constant feeling of worry or anxiety

~ Fixating on things that are outside of your control

~ Feeling mentally exhausted

~ Experiencing frequent negative thoughts, e.g. "Why do bad things always happen to me?"

~ Replaying a situation in your mind

~ Second-guessing your decisions

~ Worrying about the future

If this sounds like you, don't panic! You can break free from this negative thought spiral – you'll just need a little patience and some tips to help you look at life's challenges in a more positive way.

I can make my thoughts work in my favour

Why am I overthinking?

Sometimes we manage to convince ourselves that dwelling on a problem will help us to find the solution. Solving problems requires us to redirect our attention away from the outside world and what's going on around us in order to use our minds. And if it's a tricky problem we can get stuck inside our heads for too long. Then, as a result, we start to ignore and neglect our external environment. Before you know it, your "helpful" brain has put you into overthinking mode because that's the only way it knows how to solve a difficult or new challenge.

Here are some reasons we overthink:

~ You're feeling depressed and hopeless, which is triggering a cycle of overthinking.

~ You're being indecisive – you might be procrastinating or not looking at a problem from every angle.

~ You're struggling with low self-esteem, stress or anxiety – all can cause you to question your decisions, meaning that you overthink both the problem and a potential solution.

The negative thought cycle

If you're having a difficult day and start to overthink your worries, it's all too easy to fall into a negative thought cycle, which looks a little like this:

Negative thoughts triggered by a problem

Lack of action means the problem remains unresolved

You're overwhelmed so you start to overthink, which prohibits action

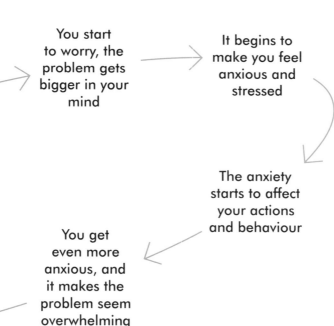

You start to worry, the problem gets bigger in your mind

It begins to make you feel anxious and stressed

The anxiety starts to affect your actions and behaviour

You get even more anxious, and it makes the problem seem overwhelming

Overthinking can take a toll on your mental well-being, so one of the best (and kindest) things we can do for ourselves is to develop ways in which we can break out of destructive thought patterns before they begin to take over.

If you run into a wall, don't turn around and give up. Figure out how to climb it.

Michael Jordan

2
Breaking the Negative Thought Cycle

Negative thoughts can be overwhelming, so it's little wonder we struggle to overcome our worries when we have a head full of negativity to contend with. And if we're overthinking all those negative thoughts too, things can quickly spiral out of control.

Life can be unpredictable. Sometimes that's good, but, other times maybe not so good. But while we can't always control what life has in store for us, we can learn some skills to help us cope when things get tough. Read on for a variety of tips and techniques to help catch those negative thoughts before they lead to overthinking.

Negative thoughts are normal

We all carry a little negativity around with us. It's practically impossible to spend all day, every day floating on your own personal cloud of happiness when you have a deadline looming or a toddler providing a soundtrack that is making your brain hurt. So it's important to recognize that negative thoughts are a typical experience for all of us – and they aren't something that can be solved with positive thinking alone. The aim is to stay realistic, recognize that you are human, and to remain hopeful during the tough times. In Chapter Four, you can find lots of top tips for embracing positivity and cultivating hope and happiness.

Let the thoughts come and go

If a negative thought makes itself known in your head (normally at an incredibly inconvenient time, like the middle of the night) try to avoid telling yourself to stop thinking that way. Instead, acknowledge the thought, and then just let it go. You can even say a mental "OK, thanks" to your brain if it helps you move your thoughts on to other things. It might help to visualize the thought as a balloon floating away, slowly getting smaller and smaller, until it's just a tiny, insignificant dot. Goodbye, negative thought!

Catch, check, challenge and change

Sometimes we're so used to listening to our own negativity that we forget to stop and ask ourselves whether it's valid or not. Instead, we just accept whatever it's saying as the truth, even though it's often wildly off the mark. One of the ways we can get a better perspective on our thoughts is to use a Cognitive Behavioural Therapy (CBT) technique called Catch, Check, Challenge and Change. It works like this:

1. Catch the thought. E.g. "Everyone in my class is better than me, I'm going to fail the test."

2. Check it: are you overthinking? Do you have evidence to support the negative thought? E.g. "It's not my strongest subject. I do find it hard, but I haven't failed a test so far."

3. Challenge it: what evidence goes against it? Can you use a positive thought to challenge it? E.g. "I've practised some tests online and completed all the revision tasks we were set in class. My tutor said I was doing great."

4. Change it: can you make the thought more balanced? E.g. "I'll probably find it a challenge, and maybe I won't get top marks, but I'll know I've tried my best."

Avoid all-or-nothing thinking

Thinking in extremes makes it difficult to get a balanced perspective and accept each situation as a unique event. For example, you might convince yourself that you'll never get a job because you were rejected by the first company who interviewed you. But frequent use of words like *never*, *always* or *nothing* makes it difficult to change the negative soundtrack in your head, which then leads to overthinking. Try using words such as *often*, *occasionally* or *sometimes* to remind the brain that setbacks do happen but that they don't have to define you.

Manage your expectations

We often envisage a situation working out one way, and then something changes and it turns out quite differently to how we'd imagined. Perhaps it's a relationship that hasn't gone as planned, or an opportunity that just didn't take off. We're left disappointed and start ruminating on what *could* have been. Then we're in the overthinking danger zone. This is especially true if we've set our hearts on a positive outcome and the reality doesn't meet our expectations.

We can't predict what life has in store for us, but if we approach each situation with an open mind, we're less likely to feel disappointed if things don't go to plan. Learn to embrace the experience and live in the present moment; that way you'll find it easier to close the door to negative thoughts too.

Bring it back to the present

If we're in the grip of a negative thought cycle, and we're overthinking our worries, it can make it tricky to think clearly. We quickly become overwhelmed with thoughts, and trying to work out a solution feels impossible. But constantly thinking about our worries – those in the past and those that *may* happen in the future – can make it difficult to enjoy life right now.

At times like this it can be helpful to bring your attention back to the present, in other words, this precise moment. Not only will it direct your focus away from negativity, but it'll help reduce your anxiety and nurture a greater appreciation of all the positive things in your life. And you can start right now!

Notice your surroundings – take note of the colour of the walls, or the clarity of the sky. Does the floor have a pattern? Are there leaves blowing in the wind? Taking in everything around you makes it easier to be more present.

Take the time to acknowledge what you have now (not in the past or in the future) and appreciate all the positive aspects of your life.

Face your inner fault finder

When something goes wrong, why do we often point the finger of blame at ourselves? Sometimes it takes only the tiniest mistake for our minds to slip into a negative fault-finding mode ("You've messed up again" or "You're not smart enough to get it right"). And then once the fault finder has gained some airtime it's difficult to drown it out.

Your inner fault finder is just throwing a bunch of unhelpful thoughts at you – but that means it can be fact-checked and put under scrutiny. And, most of the time, it's not giving you facts at all.

Next time your fault finder is an unwelcome visitor in your head, and it's got you trapped in a negative thought cycle, try interrogating it with some of these questions:

~ Am I being fair to myself?

~ Is this true? Or am I exaggerating?

~ Have I based this on fact?

~ Am I *really* going to fail after one setback?

~ Am I blaming myself for something I can't control?

Out with the bad, in with the good

The biggest challenge in breaking a negative thought cycle is to try to stop it in its tracks before it has a chance to gain traction. Which is easier said than done, right?

The trick is to identify when negative thought patterns begin (often they've been triggered by something external), briefly acknowledge them, and then replace the negativity with a positive thought you already have stored in your mental toolkit.

Next time your mind starts spouting an unhelpful narrative, think about why that might be. Did something trigger it? For example, if you had just found out that you didn't quite make the grade to get on to the college course you wanted to do, you could swap this thought:

"I just knew
I would fail. Nothing
ever goes right, and now
I've ruined my entire future.
I only have myself to blame."

For this
one:

"It's not the news
I was hoping for
but I'm grateful I still have
opportunities I can explore, and
the chance to try something different.
I might even be able to resit the exams and
re-apply next year. I'm not beaten yet!"

Let us make our future now, and let us make our dreams tomorrow's reality.

Malala Yousafzai

Track your triggers

Keeping track of our negative thoughts gives us a better chance of identifying whether something or someone is triggering the cycle to begin with. Perhaps you find that you frequently worry about body image after you've been scrolling on social media, or that you often feel down after you've spent time with a particular friend or family member. Try to jot down some of these situations so that you become more aware of when you're entering an environment that causes you anxiety, and you'll find it easier to work out a strategy to reduce these triggers.

Be honest with yourself

Being honest with ourselves is tough, even when we already have an inner critic pointing out all the things we're doing "wrong". But sometimes, if we don't ask ourselves tough questions, or scrutinize our thoughts and actions, we overlook any lessons that can be learned.

Often negative thoughts are wrapped up in a complex web that is shaped by your values and beliefs; your present circumstances as well as things that happened to you in the past, and the people you surround yourself with.

An example might be dwelling on a parenting mistake and catastrophizing the outcome to justify the belief that you're the "worst parent ever". But all the time you're dwelling on what *might* have happened, you're avoiding learning the lesson of what steps you need to take so that it doesn't happen again.

Be open to asking yourself tricky questions, such as "What should I have done differently?" and show yourself patience and understanding when the answers are uncomfortable or more complicated than just a simple "worry".

See the light in the dark

Sometimes simply reminding ourselves of all the good things in the world can be enough to break the cycle of negative thoughts. That's because the quality of our thoughts, i.e. how positive we are, influences not only how we view ourselves and the world around us, but also the outcomes that life has in store for us. It's super-simple to nurture positive thoughts; why not try:

~ Playing games. Play offers fun, silliness and joy, and is a great stress-buster too. Just taking time for a simple word or strategy game on your phone provides a sense of achievement, and nothing beats the joy of accomplishment!

~ Thinking about what you want in life... and what you need to do to get it. You could try writing your thoughts in a "dreams and aspirations" journal – it'll help to keep you optimistic and will build your confidence.

~ Making positive affirmations. When you say and repeat a positive phrase to yourself, you feel motivated and it boosts your self-esteem.

~ Giving yourself a break from the day-to-day world. Disconnect from the daily grind and its demands and spend time nurturing yourself. Put your feet up, grab a cup of your favourite drink, and watch the world outside your window. Simple activities are often best for giving your body and mind a chance to feel pure joy.

Nurture your brain by reminding yourself of all the things that make life better. Make time for the things you enjoy and the people you love, but most importantly remember that we only get one life – so make the most of it!

Reframe your point of view

Our negative thought patterns are often linked to long-held beliefs about ourselves and the world around us. For instance, if you've believed since you were young that you must have a high-paying job in order to be successful, and have then, as an adult, struggled to get such a job, you'll probably begin to feel that you're a failure. But if you can identify which beliefs are causing these negative thoughts, you can also start to challenge them.

Take the time to sit with your negative thoughts for just long enough to ask yourself why you might be thinking that way and whether the belief is justified or not. Then, instead of accepting a "faulty" belief that leads you into a negative thought cycle, see it as an opportunity to think about other viewpoints that you may not have considered, such as what really makes a person a success, i.e. feeling emotionally fulfilled, enjoying positive relationships, and making a difference to other people's lives.

Put your thoughts under the microscope

You won't need an actual microscope for this one, but you will need an open mind. Just as a scientist gathers evidence, evaluates it and comes up with a conclusion that is grounded in that evidence, you can do the same with your thoughts.

For example, you might think: "My friend thinks I'm a terrible friend." Next, write down all the evidence for this thought, such as "They didn't message me back last night" or "I wasn't able to help last time they were having a bad day", etc. Then jot down all the evidence that contradicts the thought, such as "They called me back really quickly after I rang yesterday" and "They've invited me to their barbecue next week. If they really thought I was a bad friend, they probably wouldn't invite me."

Aim to come up with a more balanced perspective, such as "My friend has other friends and wants to spend time with them too. Also, they're busy working and can't always answer the phone when I call. Being patient and understanding about this makes me a good friend, not a terrible one."

Don't get hung up on "shoulds"

Having expectations of ourselves and others can be a good thing. Setting the bar that little bit higher so that we have to stretch ourselves to reach it can help us to build resilience and determination – and having expectations of other people ensures that we surround ourselves with healthy relationships.

But sometimes expectations can become so entrenched that they turn into "rules" about how we and other people should behave. For example, thinking "My friend *should* like my social media post, because I always like theirs" might be your "rule" because you believe that acknowledging each other's social media posts is a sign of a strong relationship. But this sort of fixed mindset means that when others break our "rules" we are left upset and disappointed. And when we break our *own* rules, we feel guilty. Either way, it can send even the most open-minded people into a negative thought cycle.

Instead of seeing all the "shoulds", open your mind to all the "coulds". Perhaps your friend *could* be engaged in liking your post, but they *could* simply be spending less time on social media, or *could* be busy at work. And equally, you *could* choose to accept that they have their own expectations and that these may be different to yours. And that's perfectly OK.

*I can let go
of negative
thoughts*

Don't make space for negativity

This tip is super-simple. If we have positive influences and experiences in our lives, we're more likely to have a positive mindset. So, it makes sense that if we surround ourselves with negativity, we're making it easier for negative thoughts and feelings to take hold.

The solution? Don't make space for negativity in the first place. If you always feel tense around a particular person, try to see less of them. The same goes for certain environments and situations. Removing as much negativity from your life as you can means that you'll have more room for the things that make you feel positive.

Work on your self-acceptance

No one is perfect – we all have things we would like to improve about ourselves. But if you can learn to accept yourself in your entirety, you won't be wasting time worrying and overthinking about everything you're not. Try some of these tips for starters:

~ Acknowledge the difference between you, the person, and your behaviour. Making a stupid mistake doesn't make you a stupid person, and failing at a task doesn't mean you're a failure at life.

~ Know your values. Thinking and acting in line with your values helps to strengthen a sense of identity and boost your self-respect.

~ Don't compare yourself to others. Instead, put your energy into being the best version of yourself that you can be.

~ Establish healthy boundaries at work, in your relationships, and in terms of how you divide your time – and stick to them. It's the ultimate sign of self-respect.

~ Forgive yourself. If you've made a mistake, acknowledge it and then move on. Don't use it to berate yourself further. Self-compassion is one of the kindest things we can do for ourselves.

Try incorporating some of these ideas into your daily life. You'll quickly see that next time you're in an emotional fix, self-acceptance will be there to rescue you.

Switch your focus

Negative thoughts can very quickly become overwhelming, so if we can learn to redirect our attention away from them, even if just in the short term, it can often be enough for us to re-focus our attention elsewhere. Why not call up a loved one for a chat? Or think about something that made you laugh recently? You could even visualize something that you're excited about, like an upcoming holiday. You're not trying to avoid the negative thoughts, you're just trying to interrupt them so you can address them properly when you're not so overwhelmed. Hooray for happy thoughts!

Be your own best friend

The most important relationship you'll ever have is with yourself, so be your own best friend by showing yourself some love. Treat yourself as you would a loved one, and when negative thoughts persist, respond to them in the same way you would if a friend or family member were saying them to you. Would you tell a loved one struggling with their worries that you couldn't be bothered to help them? Thought not!

Next time you're in a destructive thought cycle, show yourself a little TLC rather than giving yourself a tough time.

Change can happen

Changing our mindset takes determination and effort, and sometimes it can feel like we're getting nowhere. But know that it will happen, even if you feel that you're barely making headway. Everyone has bad days when things don't go to plan, and on these days it's even more important that we're patient with ourselves and accept that it's OK to be hacked off – life happens, whether things are going well or badly. Obstacles help us to learn and grow, so remember to embrace the mistakes and smile at the mishaps. Better days are just around the corner.

Failure is a feeling long before it becomes an actual result.

Michelle Obama

Brain overload

Do you ever have so much on your plate that you feel like your head might explode? Fortunately, that's physically impossible, but having a busy life and juggling lots of tasks everyday can make brain explosion seem very real. Too often, many of us try to think about or do too many things at once and, before we know it, our brain becomes overloaded, and we get trapped in a negative thought cycle.

If your brain feels at risk of blowing up, consider some of these easy ideas to get back some headspace:

~ Take away the temptation of mindless scrolling by turning off notifications on your phone.

~ Concentrate on your breathing and bring your mind to the present moment (see page 138).

~ Clear your mind before bed by writing a list of everything you want to accomplish the next day.

~ Avoid trying to multitask the heck out of every day. Trying to accomplish too much at once is a fast track to brain overload. Do your brain a favour by tackling one task at a time – it'll thank you for it!

Comparing leads to despairing

Be honest – how many times have you compared yourself or your life to someone else's?

The problem is that social media, reality television and the internet have given us a window into other people's lives that makes it easy for us to compare ourselves unfavourably not just to our friends and people we know but to a bunch of people we *think* we know, such as influencers and celebrities. But if we're constantly comparing our unfiltered and sometimes chaotic lives to the perfect, curated snapshots we see online, we're making it easy for dissatisfaction and resentment to take up residence in our brains.

If you're thinking, "Why can't I be like Claire? She's always so *together*" or "I wish I was as successful as Sanjay; he can afford three holidays a year", then you need to stop right now and remember that we're all different. We all live different lives, which means our challenges and obstacles will be different too. Your life is yours, and theirs is theirs. It may not be glamorous and involve luxury yachts, but it's yours and it's authentic, so stop trampling on it with negativity and start treasuring it.

Coping with catastrophizing

Sometimes we're so caught up in our negative thoughts that we start to believe we're doomed, even in the most minor of incidents. For instance: "I've emailed the wrong person, I'll get fired" or "I haven't heard from Andy, he must have had a terrible accident", and so on ad infinitum.

This kind of negative thought spiral easily leads to overthinking. So, next time you start magnifying a problem, take a moment to stop and consider the likelihood of the "bad thing" happening – chances are it won't. You can then breathe a sigh of relief and replace the thought with a realistic one instead.

You may not control all the events that happen to you, but you can decide not to be reduced by them.

Maya Angelou

Stop trying to predict the future

Negative thinking can disguise itself as fortune telling. No, not of the mystical kind, but the kind that makes us think that we can predict the future, i.e. "I might as well give up on this essay, since I'm going to fail anyway."

Keep an open mind about what the future has in store for you. Having a set of negative expectations might feel like a safety net that allows you to cope with disappointment – but not when they become a self-fulfilling prophecy. Negative expectations also rule out opportunities for making positive changes to your life, which is crucial for your well-being.

3
Declutter Your Mind

Hands up if you frequently feel like your head is a repository for the mental junk you accumulate every day.

Whether it's worrying about something that happened last week or battling the never-ending to-do list, if you feel like your mind is constantly racing and you're overthinking all the jumbled-up thoughts in your brain it can make it difficult to focus on what's important in the here and now. If this sounds familiar, it might be time for a mental declutter – after all, there's nothing more satisfying than a good clear-out.

The write approach

Just like a messy cupboard, our minds need tidying up every now and again. But unlike the contents of a cupboard, we can't physically reorder our thoughts into neat little stacks. So we need to do the next best thing: externalize them by writing them down.

Thoughts can be difficult to catch if we're holding on to a lot of mental clutter, but if we capture them in a journal then they're not going anywhere. Jotting them down gives us a chance to offload, thereby freeing up space so we can clear our heads and find the solutions to our problems. Better still, all you need is a pen and a notepad or journal.

Journaling top tips

1. There are no "right" or "wrong" things to write down – just let your brain do the talking and you do the writing.

2. Keep going for as long as it takes to offload.

3. Reflect on what you've written – can you think of any practical solutions to your worries?

4. Try using some of the tips in Chapter One to challenge your worries – can you reframe a thought? Is there a different way of looking at it?

Small steps = big results

Picture this: you've decided to spring clean your entire house, all in one go without stopping. But the task seems so overwhelming that it paralyzes you to the point of inaction. You're not even sure how to start, let alone which room to prioritize, and suddenly the whole idea seems infeasible. So you quit, which might leave you feeling like a failure.

The same is true with our brains. Whether you're attempting to declutter your house or your mind, the same rules apply. Just tackle one room at a time – or, in the case of your mind, one small step at a time. Perhaps you want to find more time for the things that make you happy. Or you're committed to establishing some new, healthy habits. Whatever you're hoping to achieve, attempting a massive mental overhaul all at once is likely to end badly. Just take it at a pace that suits you. For example, why not try writing down some of your worries first, and start by tackling the one that's bothering you the most rather than trying to solve all of them at once. Keep it simple and enjoy the process. After all, your mind isn't going anywhere, so what's the rush?

The negativity bias

Half the time, our minds are full of thoughts that serve no purpose. Alongside all the fleeting but functional stuff like "What's for dinner?", "I should empty the bin" and "What's that smell?", we're also tuned in to background negativity, like gossipy social media posts (aka "doomscrolling") or irritating comments from a grumpy colleague, as well as our own negative self-talk. This is because as humans we're programmed to register negative stimuli more readily than positive stimuli in what psychologists call the "negativity bias".

This means that we tend to:

~ Recall traumatic experiences better than positive ones.

~ Remember insults better than we remember praise.

~ Have a stronger reaction to negative stimuli than positive stimuli.

~ Dwell on negative things more frequently than positive ones.

~ Have a stronger response to negative events than we do to equally positive ones.

If we pay more attention to the bad things that happen, it can make them seem much more important than they really are. And if your mind is trained on what's going wrong, you'll find further evidence in your life to back that up.

Try reframing the situation and look for positives instead, such as what you can learn from it, and if you find yourself ruminating, distract your brain by engaging with an activity that brings you joy.

If you can learn to let go of thoughts that don't serve you, you'll be freeing up space for positive thoughts instead.

Meditate into the moment

Get into the moment with meditation. If you're an overthinker, your mind probably spends a lot of time either rehashing the past or trying to predict future events, meaning you miss all the good stuff that's happening right now. Notice when you are worrying, or ruminating, and help your brain clear out those thoughts by meditating yourself into the present moment.

Try this:

1. Set aside 5 minutes in your day – set a timer if you need to.

2. Find a quiet, comfortable spot, free of distractions.

3. Take a breath and invite your mind to be in the present. Acknowledge any mental clutter but let go of those thoughts with your outward breath.

4. Tune into your breathing, feeling each breath in your lungs and the rise and fall of your chest.

5. If your mind wanders, simply bring it back by refocusing on your breath.

6. Finish by stretching your body and enjoying a calm moment of positivity and gratitude.

Value your values

What values do you use to define yourself? If our minds are cluttered with negative thoughts, it's often difficult to keep our focus on the things that are important to us. But knowing our personal values helps to shape the way we think, feel and behave, as well as inspiring us. Identify four core values for yourself (e.g. compassion, a sense of community, integrity, strong work ethic, etc.) and use them to help you focus your priorities and guide you down a path that's right for you.

Declutter your surroundings

Even if you're super-organized, you've probably got one area of your life that could use a little streamlining. Whether it's getting on top of general life admin or tackling the junk cupboard in the kitchen (aka the "cupboard of doom"), doing something productive to reorganize your environment doesn't just enhance your living space but can help you find some mental headspace too. If you need motivating, stick on your favourite music and just spend 10 minutes a day on your decluttering quest until you're done.

Digital detox

We've all become attached to our gadgets over the last two decades, and it's easy to see why – they help improve our productivity, make our lives easier, and save us time. What's not to love? The problem is, they often do the exact opposite.

When did you last switch off your phone? How long have you spent aimlessly scrolling today? Our digital tools are a fun distraction, but they also fill our brains with mindless thoughts. Give your brain a break by doing a one-hour digital detox. You can always try longer if you find it helps.

The worry window

If you're a perennial overthinker, it can be tough to break the habit. But what if you knew you had a window of time to worry away guilt-free?

Some overthinkers find a worry window helps them to confine their moments of angst to one small chunk of time, rather than allowing them to take over their day. Try it by scheduling a daily 15-minute worry window. If you catch yourself worrying outside of the window, just remind your brain that it's not the right time yet. Once you've reached the window you'll find that you've got a clearer head, which will allow you to start working through your worries and coming up with some solutions.

Be guided by your goals

"Goal setting" sounds a bit scary. Not only does it sound like those painful (and probably mind-numbingly dull) work appraisals, but it smacks of accountability, which comes with the added pressure to succeed.

But know this: setting some goals can be incredibly helpful – be that at work, in the home, in leisure time or in relationships. Goals help you to stay focused on what's important and stop you from getting distracted by what isn't – which is crucial if you're an overthinker and have a head full of unhelpful thoughts.

Start now by setting yourself a mini goal that's easily achievable and well within your reach. It could be anything, from clearing out that messy kitchen cupboard (see page 67) to tidying up your sock drawer. When you've gained confidence that you CAN achieve a goal, go for something bigger that's in line with your values (see page 66). Goal setting helps us to stay on track when things get tough, as well as providing a focus when our brains are overloaded – so what are you waiting for? Ready, set, goal!

Golden goals

Now that you've got a set of goals (go you!), you can put your mental energy into achieving them. Just remember these top tips:

~ Be persistent. Finish what you set out to do and you'll be proving to yourself that you can accomplish anything if you put your mind to it.

~ Don't be so hyper-focused that you close off your mind to alternative solutions. Instead, be open to reflecting regularly on your goals and changing your tactics if you need to.

~ Tell a trusted friend or loved one about your goal in order to make it "real". If it's out there in the world then you'll be accountable for achieving it. They will also make a handy cheerleader if you're flagging.

~ Focus on the outcome – you've got this!

Decide, don't deliberate

Decluttering expert and professional organizer Scott Roewer once said that "Clutter is simply delayed decisions". When you constantly deliberate, your brain quickly becomes overwhelmed by the clutter that a pending decision generates.

Whether you're putting off a difficult phone call or delaying a project that you should have started already, procrastination can use up valuable mental energy and headspace. And you could be using that space for better (and more positive) things. If you struggle with deliberation, it's time to act! Ask yourself why you're putting something off. Chances are that it's because you anticipate finding the task difficult or overwhelming. Now ask yourself whether putting it off would make the task any easier. The answer is most likely to be no – and in some cases it might even make it harder. So what are you waiting for? Just decide!

Share the load

Sometimes simply talking to a loved one about what's on your mind is enough to clear some headspace and release any pent-up emotions. Sharing your thoughts with someone you trust can also give you a fresh perspective and help you consider things from a different point of view, which can help you make better decisions.

Talking doesn't need to be tricky

If you find confiding in people difficult, it might help to write down what you want to say in advance. You could even write to them in a letter, email or text if a face-to-face chat feels too hard. Whether you're planning to meet in person or not, remember to make it clear if you just want a listening ear, or, indeed, if you'd welcome some advice.

I can let go of all distractions and fully embrace the present moment

Take a break

Taking time to unwind every day should be at the top of everyone's priority list, but it often slips to the bottom. Life is hectic, and if we're juggling multiple commitments as well as looking out for our loved ones, we tend to convince ourselves that taking time off for ourselves is somehow selfish (which it isn't, by the way...).

But your brain needs to rest and recharge so that you're clear-minded enough to tackle life's challenges. Because if you don't rest your brain, you'll be in no fit state to tackle anything! So, try switching off your phone or tablet for the ultimate relaxing experience, and just do whatever makes you feel happy. Whether it's taking a walk in the park, gardening, painting or reading a book – if it boosts your positivity, and gives you a sense of inner peace, then it's going to improve your well-being.

Try using your autopilot

Small daily tasks, like choosing what to have for breakfast or deciding what to wear, can occupy lots of brain space. It's not that it's difficult – there are just a lot of them!

Try saving some mental energy by creating a routine that you go through on autopilot. For example, have cereal for breakfast on Mondays, toast on Tuesdays, fruit on Wednesdays, and so on.

It's not a strategy that works for everyone, especially if you like a little more variety in life, but if you find that making choices about minutiae is hogging brain space, then it's worth a try!

I am in charge of how I feel today, and I choose to feel happy

Information overload

Every day we face an onslaught of information. Whether it's from newspapers, magazines, television, social media or surfing the web – the sheer quantity of information our brains digest daily can be completely overwhelming. And if we use our smartphones during the day, we're often consuming information without even seeking it out – it's simply there!

If information overload is clogging up your brain, try the following to create space:

~ Use an app that sets a limit on the amount of time you spend on social media sites or on mindlessly scrolling the internet.

~ Turn off notifications on non-essential apps. Be strict: do you really need the same news bulletin from three different outlets?

~ Unsubscribe from any blogs or e-newsletters that are not contributing to your well-being.

~ Unfollow any influencers that don't align with your core values and follow those that do.

~ Decide what information is relevant to you and your life and ignore everything else!

Picture a peaceful mind

Visualization is a powerful tool that we should all have in our decluttering armoury. If we can create a picture in our minds of what a clutter-free mind looks like, there's no reason we can't achieve it. Sounds simple, doesn't it? That's because it is! It's like daydreaming, but with a purpose. Here's how to try it:

~ Find a space where you feel relaxed and comfortable, and won't be disturbed.

~ Close your eyes and focus your attention on your breathing.

~ Imagine how a peaceful, clutter-free mind looks and feels – perhaps it resembles a clear blue sky or feels as light as a feather or weightless.

~ Imagine this state of mind manifesting into your reality.

Remember: although it might feel a bit strange and awkward the first few times you try it, it does get easier with practice. The great news is you don't need any fancy devices to give it a go – just a quiet spot and an open mind.

Empty your mind with exercise

Finding a physical activity you enjoy can be transformative. The benefits of exercising for physical and mental well-being are well documented – it helps you to stay healthy, it's a brilliant mood-booster, and it's fantastic for releasing tension and stress. If you commit to making it a daily habit, it also helps to create a sense of focus and purpose – which is exactly what you need if you're trying to reduce mental clutter.

The even better news is that you don't need to spend tons of money on a swanky gym membership (although you can if you want to) because all you really need to do is move – and that's it! Something as simple as going for a brisk walk can be just as beneficial as a session on the cross trainer. Or why not stick on your favourite playlist and dance like no one's watching? Even doing some energetic chores can count, like cleaning the windows or decluttering the attic, as does raking up leaves and mowing the lawn. You could also follow some chair-based exercises if you struggle with mobility.

The takeaway is this – if you're moving, in a way that works for you, you're doing it right.

Eliminate to accommodate

Try this super-simple tip that you can do today:

Identify any commitments that you don't need in your life. For example, you volunteered to be on the college council, but now that you're doing exams it has added extra stress you don't need. Or maybe you're on a committee at work, but it's unpaid and you have to stay late for meetings – which means that you miss valuable family time. Any activities or obligations that no longer bring you joy should be in the firing line for elimination, which will free up time and energy for the things that really matter.

When you lose you get up, you make it better, you try again.

Serena Williams

A space of your own

Humans are hardwired to be empathetic – we pick up on the moods and emotions of those around us, and this has helped us to survive as a species. But if we're unable to get away every now and again to recharge our batteries, we can find our own stress and anxiety levels rising.

To combat this, try creating a space in your home you can escape to when you're feeling overwhelmed by your thoughts. It doesn't need to be a whole room, just a quiet corner with a comfortable beanbag or chair where you can relax.

The trick is to make it a designated space, specifically for resting your mind and getting some peace and quiet – so that means no clutter and, ideally, no phones, tablets or computers either. When you feel the need to clear your head, you can retreat to this space for some much-needed downtime.

Schedule in some self-care

Self-care isn't self-indulgent – it's essential for well-being. The problem is we often feel guilty taking time off for ourselves, particularly if we've got work commitments or we're looking after a family. But taking time out to do the things we love, whether on our own or with others, is a fantastic way to clear the mind of negative thoughts.

Whether it's a gym class, reading a book or participating in your hobby, make sure each day has an activity that brings you joy scheduled in – even if it's just for 10 minutes. You can discover more self-care ideas in Chapter Four.

Set your boundaries

Setting boundaries to protect your mental space is just as important as creating a physical space you can retreat to when you're feeling overwhelmed (see page 88). Having clear emotional boundaries might mean saying no when someone asks you to do something that falls outside your schedule or doesn't align with your core values – but it'll protect your mind from the clutter of unwanted negativity.

Remember, boundaries work best when you're confident about what's OK and what's not OK for you and you can communicate it clearly to those around you. Try these boundary-setting basics to get you started:

~ Know what you want to achieve by setting a boundary, e.g. reducing demands on your time.

~ Be clear about your wants and needs – spend some time thinking about what's important to you and be prepared to express it confidently.

~ Your boundaries don't have to be fixed – you can change them at any time because you're in charge.

~ Don't forget to set boundaries with yourself too – such as knowing when to take time out if you're overthinking.

~ Remember to respect other people's boundaries just as you respect your own.

Embrace being imperfect

Perfect doesn't exist, so it's totally irrational that we waste valuable headspace stressing over it. No one is perfect and there is no such thing as perfect – got it? The problem is, we tend to obsess over the idea of being perfect – perfect body, perfect job, perfect lifestyle and so on – but really we ought to be letting go of this type of damaging thought and embracing our imperfections instead. Learn to be kinder to yourself and let go of any unrealistic expectations that don't serve you in a positive way.

Lighten the load

If your mind is like a huge list of things to do, it might be time to delegate some tasks to a loved one. This is particularly true if you're a parent or carer and you're carrying the mental load on behalf of everyone. There's a strong chance that your loved ones do not realize that you're struggling – and will be happy to help lighten the load once they know that you are.

Once you begin to delegate tasks, you'll probably experience not only a huge sense of relief but also a sense of freedom from the burden of responsibility, leading to more time and headspace for positive things instead. Result!

Forgive and forget

Often our minds feel cluttered because we're carrying around guilt and regret from the past, along with a host of other negative emotions that no longer serve us. It's a little like dragging around a suitcase full of clothes we no longer wear and things we don't need! If we can learn to let go of these unhelpful thoughts, by forgiving ourselves, it can help to reduce the clutter in our minds and to nurture a sense of inner peace. Only then can we really grow and move forward in life.

Self-forgiveness does not mean condoning your behaviour or letting yourself off the hook. It signifies that you accept what has happened, and the behaviour that prompted it, and are willing to move on without ruminating over something that can't be changed.

Remember these key steps next time you need to forgive yourself:

~ Accept **responsibility** for your actions and show compassion to yourself.

~ Show **remorse** for what happened without being self-critical. Instead be compassionate and acknowledge that you made a mistake and want to do better in the future. Guilt can serve as a motivator for positive behaviour change.

~ **Restore** the relationship with yourself and anyone else you may have hurt by rectifying your mistakes and apologizing if necessary.

~ **Reflect** on what you can learn from the experience and how you can use that knowledge and experience to guide your actions in the future.

~ **Renew** your faith in yourself by committing to making better choices in the future.

Break it down

Sometimes we get so overwhelmed we don't even know where to start – and then we start overthinking the fact that we're overwhelmed and don't know where to start! This can cause a great deal of clutter to accumulate, but using some basic time-management techniques can help to alleviate it.

Simply write down any tasks that need to be completed in order of priority. Then break them into smaller chunks and give each of them a time frame. Then focus on completing each task, one at a time. Resist the temptation to multitask or you'll start collecting clutter again. Then, once you're done, reward yourself with something fun so that you celebrate your new organizational skills!

Faith is taking the first step, even when you don't see the whole staircase.

Martin Luther King Jr

Don't be everyone's problem-solver

Are you the person everyone comes to when they've got a problem? Kudos to you – this means that you're an excellent problem-solver (and no doubt an awesome friend too), but sometimes carrying the burden of not only your own issues but everyone else's can be completely overwhelming. Especially if those troubled people aren't prepared to make changes or to solve problems themselves.

The solution? Learn to let go of what you can't control – you're not their personal problem-solver. Only they can change the outcomes in their lives. You're their friend out of choice, not because they're a drama llama who needs someone to hold their hand. Be supportive, yes, but if you're constantly worrying on their behalf and they're not taking steps to help themselves, then it might be time to rethink your boundaries, or even to step away from the relationship entirely.

Take time to ground yourself

If we're constantly busy and juggling multiple thoughts, it doesn't take much to tip us over the edge and into the overthinking zone. It's at such times that taking a break to calm and clear the mind of any worries should be a top priority, and this can be done by grounding ourselves in the present – a technique that helps to steer the mind away from negative or challenging emotions.

Try this next time you're overwhelmed and it's making you anxious:

The 5-5-5 game

Take a deep breath. Look around the room and name five things that you can see aloud. Now close your eyes and take another breath, then name five things you can hear. You can reopen your eyes if you want to or keep them closed.

Take another breath. Now name five body parts and move them in turn, e.g. say "toes" and then wriggle your toes. Go back to the beginning of the exercise and keep doing all the steps until a sense of calm is restored.

Watch your language

You are not your problems, and you're also not your failures. Yet we frequently convince ourselves that we *are* the problem because of the language we use when we're in dialogue with ourselves (i.e. our thoughts). For us to gain perspective and realize that our worries don't define us, we need to reframe how we talk to ourselves.

Instead of thinking, "I'm an overthinker", replace that thought with "I'm noticing that I'm overthinking." Doing this will help you separate your challenges from your sense of identity and self-worth – meaning you'll stop blaming yourself every time you become overwhelmed by negative thoughts.

Acceptance

If you want to live without the burden of negativity, just remember this: learn to accept the things you can't change but aim to change the things you can't accept. Know that the more you can change the things in your life that you refuse to accept, such as being around negative people, or allowing yourself to have unhealthy habits, the more resilient you will become, and the less cluttered your mind will be.

Only you are the master of your mind, so start accepting the path you're on – just make sure it's the right one for you.

Mental minimalism

As we've discovered, we exist in an information-rich world, which can often distort what we *think we want* as opposed to what we *actually need* to live a happy and fulfilled life. We get confused about what we should want, especially if other people want different things for us, creating an imbalance around our expectations of ourselves and the expectations of others. We can also be swayed by what we believe society expects of us, perhaps from social media, influencers, and a whole host of other fleeting impulses that, when you drill down, are pretty superficial and don't serve us at all. Little wonder our brains get cluttered.

Try practising mental minimalism. It's a way of recognizing what's truly important and significant to you and deciding if those things contribute to your life so that you can achieve peace of mind. True needs are mostly felt and expressed simply and explicitly – like hugging the person you love. Let the memories of those moments take up brain space rather than worrying about the latest gimmick or buying a product just because an influencer told you to. Keep life simple – cuddle the cat or go for a walk with a loved one. Play a silly game with the kids or call a friend you haven't spoken to in a while. If it gives you a little boost of happiness, you're on the right track.

You're in the driving seat

Now that you've had a good decluttering, it's time to look forward and work out what direction you're heading in so you can make the most of your time and energy. Life will always try to throw time-hogging obstacles at you – and nothing will change that – but now that you've got some clarity of thought, you can start to structure your life so you're doing more of what matters and less of what doesn't.

To get a better balance, you could try the following:

1. Decide on the three values or priorities that matter most to you.

2. Keep a note of how you spend your time every day in as much detail as you can, for example, "15 minutes on social media, 10 minutes on a call", etc.

3. Analyze the data: is your time reflecting your values? How are you spending most of your time? And the least amount of time?

4. Restructure your time to better reflect your values. For example, if one of your values is prioritizing family time, you might need to change your work pattern.

5. After a few weeks reflect on whether your new structure is working out or not and adjust it if necessary.

Seeking help

Sometimes, those with an underlying condition such as depression, anxiety or attention deficit hyperactivity disorder (ADHD), can find it especially challenging to cope with an overloaded mind. If you're feeling overwhelmed to the point where you're struggling to function normally in your daily life, it might be time to seek professional help. There is a list of organizations at the end of this book that can provide help and advice, alongside speaking to your doctor or healthcare provider.

The past is the past,
it doesn't predict
my future

Happiness cannot come from without. It must come from within.

Helen Keller

4

Embrace
Positive Thinking

Nurturing a positive attitude is one of the kindest things you can do for yourself. In fact, it's the ultimate expression of self-love! Positive thinking can help you overcome adversity, encourage resilience, and increase feelings of joy and happiness – all of which will also help you to overcome your overthinking.

It won't be a quick fix. Just like building up muscles in the gym, you need to retrain your mental muscles to seek out the positives rather than absorb the negatives. This can be particularly challenging if you struggle with anxiety and depression, but if you aim to start small, and give yourself time to grow, you'll be practising positivity already!

Practise gratitude

Expressing gratitude to someone, or for something, is one of the simplest, but most effective ways to nurture positivity in our lives. When we've got a lot going on inside our heads, it's difficult to remember all the wonderful things in our lives. Showing gratitude reminds us that even among the chaos of an overthinking mind, we still have things to be thankful for.

Take a few moments each day to write down a few things you're grateful for. It could be something small, like being thankful for a sunny day, or something bigger such as having an amazing partner and friends. This will help ground you and keep your mind calm and ready to focus on the positives rather than getting clogged up with negatives.

Do something kind

When our minds are cluttered by overthinking, we tend to go into ourselves. We focus on our own worries, and they become all-consuming, often to the detriment of the people around us.

But there's an easy fix for this that'll not only make you feel more positive but will spread positivity to those around you too. And it's this – do something kind for someone else. It will help you divert the focus away from your worries and on to something positive, as well as giving your mind the breathing space it needs to tackle your own challenges head-on with renewed optimism.

*I'd rather regret
the risks that
didn't work out
than the chances
I didn't take at all.*

Simone Biles

Nurture positivity with nature

Being in nature can really help to nurture those positive vibes and our overall well-being. It helps us to reconnect with ourselves and regain clarity of mind – and having a clear mind is crucial for overcoming overthinking. Not only that, being in nature helps to reduce stress, increase energy levels, and elevate fitness levels. And, if that's not convincing enough, studies have consistently shown that being in nature reduces feelings of isolation, promotes a sense of calm and lifts mood – hurrah for nature!

Aim to escape into the great outdoors every day if you can. Explore the local park, woods, riverside walks or coastline, and if you can't leave the house, you can bring nature in with house plants or by growing flowers on the windowsill. Growing salad plants, vegetables and herbs is also a great option, with the added benefit of providing a healthy source of food for you and your friends and family to enjoy.

People power

The people we surround ourselves with can have a significant impact on the way we think and how we feel, so it's important to ensure that we've got positive, supportive and encouraging individuals in our lives who will lift us up rather than drag us down.

Positive relationships help to reduce mental clutter and stress because, if you're secure in your relationships, you're less likely to spend time worrying and overthinking them. Spend some time evaluating who you spend your time with – do they bring out the best in you? Have they got your back even when times are tough? Toxic relationships can cause negativity, as well as feelings of self-doubt and anxiety, so it's important to identify these relationships, put healthy boundaries in place, and, if necessary, learn how to let them go.

Ending a relationship the "healthy" way

Ending any relationship is tough, but knowing how to do it well can help make it less harmful for all involved. To give both sides the best chance, you should:

1. Acknowledge that it may cause pain for both of you.

2. Always have a face-to-face conversation.

3. Be honest but don't go into tiny details.

4. Avoid arguing and raised voices.

5. Make a clean break, at least in the short term – some distance and time for reflection will aid healing.

6. Try not to shame or blame the other person.

7. Give yourself time to grieve the end of the relationship.

If you're finding the behaviour of a close friend or family member challenging but it isn't possible to end the relationship entirely, try minimizing the contact you do have and try to ensure that other people are there to act as a "buffer" if you are in their company.

Getting enough sleep

When we're well rested we feel invincible! Well... almost. But it's a proven fact that a regular sleep routine is key to keeping our mental and physical well-being in tip-top condition. Getting adequate sleep helps reduce stress levels and improves our concentration, which helps us to function in our waking hours and be ready to take on whatever life has in store for us that day.

Sleep 101

~ Aim for seven to nine hours of quality sleep each night. If you find it hard to get into the sleep zone, try meditation or do a brain-dump into a journal to help clear your head.

~ Stash away your devices at least one hour before bed so that you're not churning information around your head when it hits the pillow.

~ Try to set your body clock by going to sleep at the same time every night – try not to nap during the afternoon or evening or you'll be up until the small hours!

~ Fresh air and exercise ensure the best night's sleep so try to include both in your daily routine.

Affirmations

Our minds are powerful, so let's use some of that power to generate positivity! We've already seen how our minds can learn to reframe negative thoughts, and affirmations are an extension of that. The idea is that if you affirm something positive to yourself repeatedly, your brain will start to believe it, such as "I love myself just as I am", and "I am proud of myself for trying."

Affirmations can have a significant impact on how we view ourselves and the world around us, and if used regularly can help to train your mind to focus on positivity.

I have everything I need to achieve my goals

Be your own cheerleader

We all have times when we feel like we're flagging. Perhaps you've got lots on at work, or multiple commitments that need to be fulfilled and it feels like you're getting nowhere. Or maybe you're simply drained from the demands of looking after a family.

It's at times like this that it becomes hard to keep up your momentum and to stay positive, so when you start to feel this way, why not try giving yourself a pep talk? You can either say it aloud or in your head, but the aim is for it to inspire you to stay positive when things get tough.

What if?

Try to visualize what your life would look like if your perspective was more positive. Would you actively seek out new opportunities? Would you have the resilience to overcome your overthinking and tackle life's challenges?

Visualizing what we could achieve if we encourage positivity into our lives is a bit like a mental rehearsal for living it out in real life. Your mind is your most powerful ally, so use it to your advantage by imagining positive outcomes for your life goals – and then use that insight to make it a reality!

Healthy body, healthy brain

Keeping our bodies physically healthy helps our minds to stay healthy too – so it's the ultimate act of self-care. Exercise releases lots of helpful mood-boosting neurotransmitters called endorphins, which make us feel more positive about ourselves and the world around us. They also help to reduce anxiety and boost energy and confidence levels.

So, we know the science – but what about putting it into practice? Maybe you've got regular exercise nailed and it's one of your favourite things to do (go you), but there's also a possibility that just reading this is making you want to weep. And that's OK too! If the thought of exercising sounds more painful than pleasurable, you need to choose an activity you want to do, rather than those you think you should do. Consider the physical activities you enjoyed as a child – could you turn your nostalgia for those into a new fitness hobby?

If you need some inspiration, you could try:

Skipping

Hula-hooping

Pilates

Table tennis

Adult gymnastics

Yoga

Rowing or kayaking

Skateboarding

In-line skating

Dance classes

Cycling

Jogging or running

Walking or hiking

Swimming

Gardening

Get up and go!

Being positive is all about taking action, rather than watching the action pass you by. It's about knowing you've got the get-up-and-go to enjoy life to the full and using your energy and drive to tackle life's challenges. It doesn't have to be hard work either, often the simplest acts have the most positive effect on mindset.

Next time you need a positivity boost, consider taking action in one of these ways:

~ Listen to your favourite music – whether it's reggae, classical, folk music or anything else, belting out some tunes is a fantastic way to encourage positivity.

~ Engage with activities that give you good vibes, like meditation, playing a sport, or spending time on your hobby.

~ Just smile! Smiling releases endorphins and gives you an instant shot of nature's good stuff. If you're having the day from hell, try listening to a funny podcast or watching your favourite upbeat movie to get the feel-good chemicals flowing again.

~ Write some affirmations for yourself on slips of paper and put them in a jar. Do a lucky dip every morning and use the affirmation throughout the day to inspire you.

Self-care = self-love

Self-care isn't selfish – it's vital! Taking time off for yourself, guilt-free, is crucial for your sense of self-worth. It ensures that you are doing all the things your body and mind need to function at their best, and helps you to live a healthy, positive life.

Anything you do for yourself that makes you feel happy is self-care, like spending an extra hour in bed so you're fully rested, getting some exercise, or baking a cake and sharing it with your family. The rule of thumb is this: if it gives you confidence, inner peace and improves your well-being, then you're on the right track.

I love and accept myself, always

Eat well to live well

If we fuel our bodies with all the nutritious delicious goodness that we can, we'll be fuelling our minds too. That's because if our bodies have energy and stamina, our brains follow suit – which gives us the best chance of staying positive and being resilient. That's why we get "hangry" if we're not eating the right foods!

According to the World Health Organization, a healthy diet for adults contains protein, fruit, vegetables, legumes (e.g. lentils and beans), nuts and whole grains (e.g. unprocessed maize, millet, oats, wheat and brown rice), as well as a few carbs and a small amount of sugar and fat.

Aim to eat three healthy meals a day, with some nutritious snacks in between.

Snacktastic tip

If you're someone who grazes then try to choose snacks that are high in vitamins and release energy slowly in order to avoid the inevitable irritability when your blood sugar levels drop! Probiotic yoghurt, an oat-and-dried-fruit cereal bar or wholewheat crackers with hummus are all good options if you need a body and brain boost.

Become a pro at positive self-talk

The dialogue we have with ourselves makes a dramatic difference to how positive we feel – especially when there's negative chatter and noise to cut through. So, we need to make sure that we're nailing it! According to psychology experts, language matters. Studies show that the best way to talk positively to yourself is to talk in the third person, by using your pronouns or name. This provides the distance needed to control thoughts, feelings and behaviour more effectively.

Here's an example:

> ### Talk the talk
>
> Humza is running a charity race, so to help motivate himself he could say this:
>
> "Humza has put the effort into his training. He is strong, energized and ready for the challenge. It means so much to him to help raise money. He crosses the line knowing he's made a difference."

Find the sweet spot

When you're feeling positive you can achieve your full potential. So, if you can find that sweet spot of joy in your life that brings you all the tingly good feels, you need to hold on to it – and preferably do more of it!

Perhaps you enjoy walking through the autumn leaves or finding shells on the beach. Maybe it's as simple as surrounding yourself with furry friends and enjoying a cuddle, or watching the sunset with a loved one. Always make time for whatever fills your heart with happiness – it's an investment you'll never regret.

Go on an adventure

Adventures don't have to stop once we're firmly into adulthood. Getting in touch with our inner child can liberate us and transport us back to those halcyon days when we were young, carefree and the sun always shone... you get the picture!

Indulging in some youthful pastimes can be great for positivity. Fly a kite or build a den in the garden. Have a water fight or go on a scavenger hunt in the woods. Reconnecting with the joy we felt as children can be a brilliant way to live joyfully as an adult.

Mindful mini-break

One of the most powerful ways you can calm a busy mind and invite positivity into your life is to practise everyday activities in a mindful way. Mindfulness involves focusing on the present moment and using your senses to ground yourself – it's a bit like taking your brain on a mini-break so that it gets a rest from all of life's distractions. It can feel a little strange to begin with, but with practice it will help you set aside your worries and make some headspace for positive thinking instead.

To give it a go, try looking at the world outside your window as though you were seeing it for the first time, like this:

1. Find your nearest window and get comfortable, either sitting or standing.

2. Give your absolute full attention to what you can see outside the window – it's your whole universe for the next minute.

3. Study everything, including colours, textures or patterns, but avoid labelling things. For instance, instead of "grass", notice the different shades of green.

4. Don't forget movement. How is the breeze blowing the tree? Or the washing on the line?

5. Are there any sounds outside? Is there a scent in the air?

Celebrate the small wins

Everyone likes to feel that they're achieving something – whether they're age five or ninety-five! And what's great is that we don't have to win a race or a competition to congratulate ourselves on a job well done – because we all achieve something, no matter how small, every day.

So don't wait for someone to start playing a fanfare – give yourself a pat on the back instead! Managed to get the kids in bed by 8 p.m.? That's worth a fist pump. Got through a tricky lesson at college? Give yourself a round of applause. By focusing on the small wins, you'll feel like you're making progress, meaning that it'll be easier for you to stay positive.

Nothing is impossible; the word itself says "I'm possible"!

Audrey Hepburn

*I am always
true to myself
and my values*

5
Next Steps

Now that you have a toolkit of tips to help you cope with an overthinking brain, it's time to think about the next steps on your well-being journey.

The future doesn't have to be scary. In fact, if you've worked your way through this book, hopefully you're starting to see that the future is bright with possibilities. Know that each step you take towards positivity is a step in the right direction – you've got this!

Good habits

Aim to establish some of your new positive thinking skills as regular habits in your daily routine. Science tells us that when we repeatedly do the same thing, as we do when we develop a habit (good or bad), it can feel comforting. The feel-good hormone, dopamine, is released in your body and you get a little boost of happiness. That's why your first slurp of a latte in the morning, and the caffeine hit that follows, is the best one of the day!

Building new, healthy habits into your routine is simple. Try these tips to get started:

~ Prep your environment – e.g. if you're planning to start your day by doing some hopeful journaling, make sure that your journal and pen are easy to find when you get out of bed.

~ Start small and remind yourself of the benefits – know why you are making the change and use it to motivate yourself.

~ Linking new habits to existing healthy habits is the best way to make them stick – e.g. tag a 10-minute meditation on to your bedtime yoga routine.

~ Do a fist pump whenever you practise your habit effectively – it'll help build a positive association.

Changing direction

Don't ever be afraid to correct your course. Sometimes overthinking can cause us to become paralyzed by the fear of change. Whether it's a minor adjustment in your life such as giving up coffee and cake for a healthier option, or a big change in circumstances such as moving to another country or taking a career break to start a family, change provides us with an amazing opportunity for personal growth.

The dreams, aspirations and hopes that we have for ourselves when we're younger very rarely translate to the lives we lead as adults. And that's not a bad thing: it's just part of the rich tapestry of life. If you need to alter your direction of travel, just do it – your life is your own, and as you grow and develop as a person you'll need to take some detours. Just be open to other possibilities and don't be scared to reroute yourself if you need to.

Bounce back

Not everything in life will go your way, so making sure that you're resilient in response to all the obstacles you'll encounter is vital to maintaining a positive outlook. The good news is that resilience is something that can be learned with a few simple rules:

Golden rules of resilience

~ Work on your self-belief – practise affirmations and surround yourself with people who lift you up.

~ See the glass as half-full; seek solutions, not problems – remind yourself of all the difficult things you've already overcome.

~ Embrace a growth mindset – see change as an opportunity and keep looking to the future rather than gazing back at the past.

Talk it out

One of the best things you can do to overcome your overthinking is to talk about it with someone close to you, whether that's a family member or a trusted friend. Being open about your worries, and how you sometimes feel overwhelmed, gives your loved ones the opportunity to provide support and assistance. If you've surrounded yourself with people who value you, they'll be only too happy to lend a hand – just as you would for them.

If you go through life believing that happiness is somewhere in your future, it always will be.

Steven Bartlett

Seeking professional help

If you're feeling so overwhelmed with worry that you're struggling to function normally in your daily life, it might be time to seek professional help. You should always speak to your doctor or healthcare provider for advice before accessing support from other organizations.

Samaritans (UK)
Freephone 116 123
www.samaritans.org
The Samaritans provide mental health support and a listening service for those who wish to speak to someone confidentially and without judgement. You can also chat to a listening volunteer online and access the Samaritans self-help app via the website.

Campaign Against Living Miserably (UK)
Freephone 0800 58 58 58
www.thecalmzone.net
CALM offers life-saving services to those who are feeling hopeless and aims to show that life is always worth living. If you're struggling, you can talk to a trained member of staff either on a call or web chat. The service is free, confidential and anonymous.

Mental Health America (US)
www.mhanational.org
The MHA website provides information on Warmlines – a number you can call in your state to access support from a trained professional when life is tough.

SANE (AUS)
1800 187 263
www.sane.org
Information and crisis support for people with mental health challenges and their families, living in Australia.

Your fabulous future

Change can be scary – fact. The decisions you're making right now will have consequences in the future, and that's quite a responsibility. But your future can, and will, be fabulous if you keep in mind these key points:

~ Don't let the past define you – acknowledge mistakes then move on.

~ Know your values and what you stand for – set boundaries if you need to.

~ Forgive and forget – life is too short to bear grudges. That includes forgiving yourself.

~ Question and interrogate your worries and negativity – are they justified? Chances are that the answer is a big NO, so don't waste energy on it!

Each new day
I wake up stronger

Conclusion

How you choose to live your life is up to you, but if you want to overcome your overthinking and make positivity your goal – don't give up! You can achieve anything you want by meeting obstacles head-on and by focusing on a positive outcome. Our worries should never become a factor that defines us – challenges are just part of life – but we can choose to let happiness and joy define who we are and what we stand for.

Through reading this book, hopefully you've been reassured that overthinking doesn't need to stop you from living your best life. Armed with the tips and techniques you've read about, you can live a life that honours your values, frees your mind of troubling thoughts, and lets you focus on being the best version of yourself you can possibly be. So, move forward with a calmer mind, and embrace a more positive future.

Resources

In addition to the organizations detailed on pages 150–151, you can find inspiration, ideas and support in the following resources.

Websites

www.nhs.uk/every-mind-matters (UK)
www.mind.org.uk (UK)
www.headtohealth.gov.au (Australia)
www.wellnesstogether.ca (Canada)
www.psychcentral.com (USA)

Podcasts

Calmly Coping – Self-help podcast for overthinkers who appear calm and collected on the outside, but are struggling, doubting, and overthinking on the inside.
Good Life Project – Questions and topics related to well-being, happiness and relationships are explored every week in conversation with leading voices from different fields, including health, science, the arts, business, and the wellness sector.

The Overthinker's Guide to Joy – Everyday tips and tricks on how to manage your stress and overthinking brain so you can reduce stress, improve your health and find more joy in your life.

Books

How to Worry Less: Tips and Techniques to Help You Find Calm, Claire Chamberlain (2022)
The Worry Cure: Seven Steps to Stop Worry from Stopping You, Robert L. Leahy (2005)
Stop Overthinking: 23 Techniques to Relieve Stress, Stop Negative Spirals, Declutter Your Mind, and Focus on the Present, Nick Trenton (2021)

Online forums, support groups and communities

www.dailystrength.org/group/anxiety
www.mentalhealthforum.net
www.support.therapytribe.com/anxiety-support-group

The Anxiety Fix
Gentle Exercises to Help Calm Your Mind
Anna Barnes

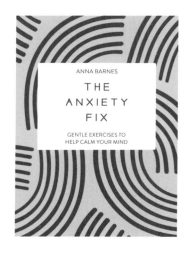

Paperback
ISBN: 978-1-83799-160-0

Quieten your mind with this guided journal, filled with practical tips and simple strategies for managing feelings of anxiety.

Anxiety can feel like a huge obstacle to living the life you want – but it doesn't have to be! Brimming with practical activities and inspiring words, *The Anxiety Fix* is a gentle and encouraging guide to help you flourish.

The Confidence Fix
Empowering Exercises to Build Your Self-Esteem

Debbi Marco

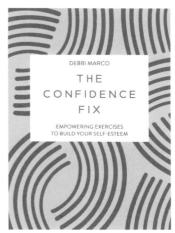

Paperback
ISBN: 978-1-83799-306-2

Embrace your inner confidence and unleash your full potential with this simple guide to boosting your self-esteem.

Confidence isn't something we are born with, but instead is a skill that can be learned and developed over time. Filled with inspiring statements and practical activities, *The Confidence Fix* is a gentle and encouraging guide on how to grow your self-assurance.